SLEEP BETTER IN 21 DAYS

Change Your SUBCONSCIOUS Blueprint to Enjoy a Good Night's Sleep

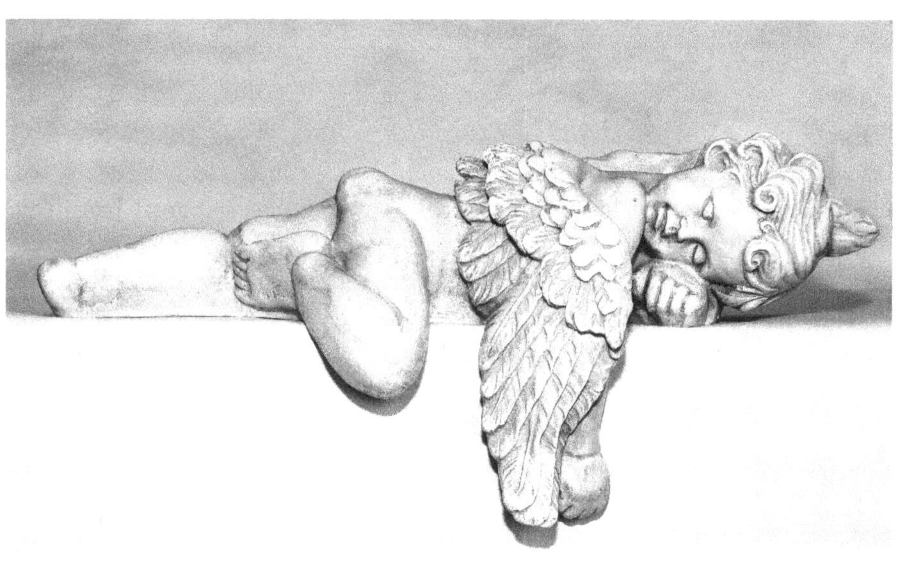

Steve Thomas GQHP

(Certified Hypnotherapist and Mind Coach)

© Copyright 2020 (Steve Thomas GQHP) - All rights reserved.
The contents of this book may not be reproduced, duplicated or transmitted without direct written permission from the author.
Under no circumstances will any legal responsibility or blame be held against the publisher for any reparation, damages, or monetary loss due to the information herein, either directly or indirectly.

Legal Notice:
This book is copyright protected. This is only for personal use. You cannot amend, distribute, sell, use, quote or paraphrase any part or the content within this book without the consent of the author. You are not authorized to share password access.

Disclaimer Notice:
Please note the information contained within this document is for educational and entertainment purposes only. Every attempt has been made to provide accurate, up to date and reliable complete information. No warranties of any kind are expressed or implied. Readers acknowledge that the author is not engaging in the rendering of legal, financial, medical or professional advice. The content of this book has been derived from various sources. Please consult a licensed professional before attempting any techniques outlined in this book.

By reading this document, the reader agrees that under no circumstances is the author responsible for any losses, direct or indirect, which are incurred as a result of the use of information contained within this document, including, but not limited to, —errors, omissions, or inaccuracies.

The photographs used in this eBook are royalty free photographs procured from various websites affiliated to Creative Commons such as Pixabay and Wikimedia commons. There are also some YouTube video links.

Table Of Contents

"The best bridge between despair and hope is a good night's sleep."
— E. Joseph Cossman

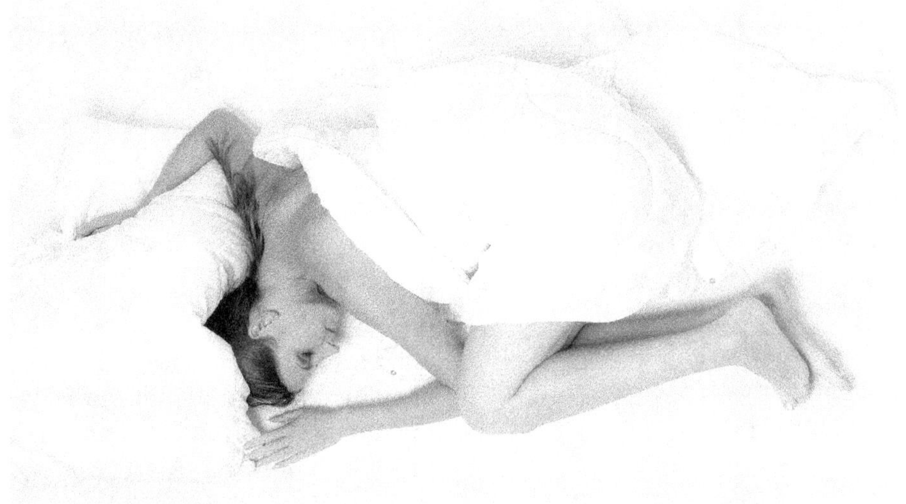

A Good Night's Sleep is essential for optimal health since it can affect your mood, weight, and hormone levels. If you suffer from sleep disorders, it can severely affect your overall well-being.

Sleep disorders can affect your ability to sleep well. Primarily caused by excess stress or an existing health problem, sleep disorders are increasingly becoming common across the globe.

According to a **study conducted in the US**[1], more than one-third of people reported getting less than 7 hours of sleep in a day. Another **study conducted on high school students**[2] in the US revealed that more than seventy percent of them reported getting less than 8 hours of sleep on school nights.

Most people typically experience sleep problems as a result of hectic schedules, stress, and other external influences. But, when these start happening on a regular basis and mess up your daily life, these may point to a sleep disorder.

If you find it difficult to fall asleep at night, this may result in an extremely tiresome mood throughout the next day. It can also adversely affect your overall health, mood, energy, and focus.

Sleep disorders can take a serious toll on your physical and mental health. Frequent sleep troubles can be a frustrating and devastating experience. It can have a negative impact on your ability to deal with stress. Ignoring sleep disorders may result in various problems such as weight gain, memory issues, impaired job performance, strained relationships, and even road mishaps.

In certain cases, sleep disorders can be a warning sign of some other mental or medical condition. Once the treatment is obtained for the root cause of your sleep disorder, this problem may eventually disappear.

You don't need to live with sleep disorders! There are multiple ways to identify the root cause of your sleep problems and improve your overall health and quality of life. My name is Steve Thomas and I am a Certified Hypnotherapist and Mind Coach.

I created this book to help hundreds and thousands of people who not only suffer from sleep disorders but also from other issues such as lack of self-confidence.

Hypnotherapy can not only help you tackle sleep disorders but can also help you achieve your desired goals and live the life you deserve by getting rid of those unwanted habits.

Whether it's a weight-loss issue, quitting smoking issue, exam nerves, anxiety, phobia, or extreme stress, hypnotherapy can definitely help guide you into an altered state of awareness. It enables your brain to process information more efficiently and in a different manner.

Hypnotherapy helps ascertain your current needs and access your subconscious to bring about unconscious change by creating new thought patterns, responses, attitudes, and behaviors.

Hypnosis is a natural state that you achieve multiple times in a day. For example, while brushing your teeth you were daydreaming of something else – you were in trance! Your thoughts were elsewhere when you got dressed for your office. While driving or traveling to work you were thinking of something else.

In fact, according to many experts, we humans live in trance 95 percent of the time. But, it doesn't matter whether or not we are in trance. What matters is whether it's a helpful or unhelpful trance. Unhelpful trance includes habits such as overeating, smoking, and constantly worrying about external things that you can't control.

Hypnotherapy can help you to create a day-dream like state in your mind and implant new thoughts and outlooks that can help improve your life for the better.

I created this book to help you from a psychological viewpoint to improve your overall physical wellbeing using a holistic approach. If you have a physical condition that is affecting your sleep, you're advised to visit your physician first. This book is not a replacement for professional medical advice.

Also, this book comes with links to HYPNOTIC AUDIOS your access password is in the reference section. To get full benefit from your free audios, I suggest you read and study this book, it's a short read, and I think an easy read. Do not listen to these hypnotic audios when driving, operating heavy machines, or carrying out any manual tasks requires your full attention.

In this book, I have done an in-depth analysis of sleep and sleep disorders, its diagnosis, and effective treatment, and tools for successful sleep so that you can readily grasp everything smoothly, fairly, and quickly!

So, without further ado,

LET'S GET STARTED!

The Importance Of Sleep

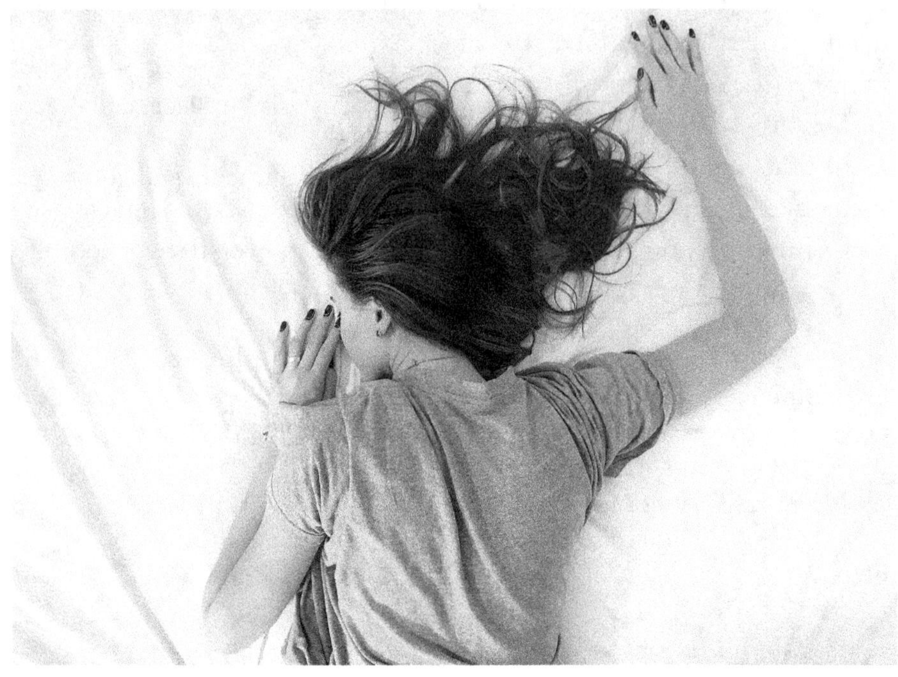

A Good night's sleep is really important for your overall physical, mental, and spiritual wellbeing. It's your important daily routine as you spend nearly 1/3rd of your time doing it.

Just like water and food, getting enough amount of quality sleep at the right times is essential for survival. Lack of sleep will inhibit the formation or maintenance of your brain pathways that allow you to create new memories and learn faster. It will be difficult for you to respond quickly and focus for a longer period.

Sleep is vital to various brain functions such as communication between neurons (nerve cells). In reality, your brain remains remarkably active during your sleep. Various studies suggest that toxins accumulate in your brain while you are awake and quality sleep helps remove those toxins from your brain.

Sleep is a dynamic and complex process and its biological purpose remains a mystery to date. Sleep affects nearly all types of system, organ, and tissue in your body — from your brain, lungs, and heart to the immune system, metabolism, and disease resistance.

Various studies revealed that poor quality sleep or a lack of sleep can increase the risk of several ailments such as cardiovascular disease, high blood pressure, obesity, depression, and diabetes.

1.1) Sleep Anatomy

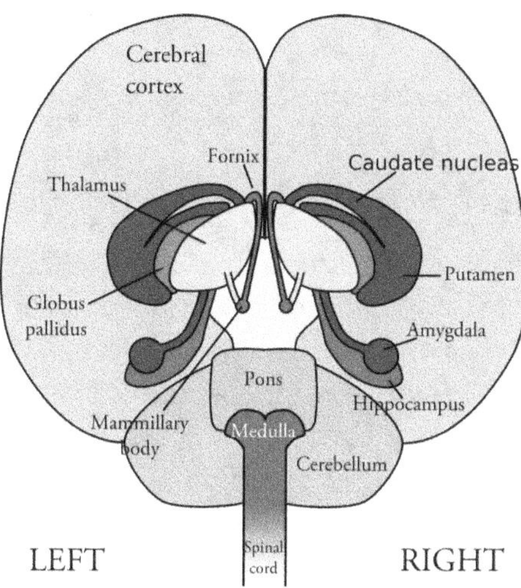

Following are the structures inside your brain that are involved while you sleep:

Hypothalamus: It's a peanut-sized structure inside your brain that holds groups of nerve cells, which work as control centers affecting arousal and sleep. Inside the hypothalamus, there is the SCN (Suprachiasmatic Nucleus) that contains clusters of thousands of cells that get light exposure information straight from your eyes and control your circadian rhythm (sleep-wake cycle). People with damaged SCN sleep irregularly during the day as they don't have the ability to manage their circadian rhythms. Most blind people possess some ability to sense light and they modify their circadian rhythm accordingly.

Brain Stem: Located at the base of the brain, the brain stem contains structures such as the midbrain, medulla, and pons. Brain stem works with the hypothalamus to control your circadian rhythm. Both contain sleep-promoting cells that produce a brain chemical known as GABA, which helps reduce the arousal activity in your brain. The pons and medulla (structures in the brain stem) play a special role in REM (rapid eye movement) sleep. These send signals to relax muscles responsible for limb movements and body posture to prevent you from acting out your dreams.

Thalamus: This structure is responsible for the communication of information between the senses and the cerebral cortex. The cerebral cortex interprets and processes information from short-term to long-term memory. Thalamus remains quiet during most stages of sleep to help you tune out the external world. However, it becomes active during the REM sleep stage and transmits the cortex images, sounds, and other feelings that fill your dreams.

Pineal gland: This structure is located in the two hemispheres of your brain. Once it receives signals from the SCN, it increases the production of melatonin hormone that helps you sleep quickly when the lights are off. Visually impaired people who cannot control their circadian rhythm using natural light can coordinate their wake-sleep patterns by having small quantities of melatonin each day at the same time.

Basal forebrain: Located near the bottom and front of the brain, the basal forebrain also promotes your circadian rhythm as well as the arousal system. The cells in the basal forebrain release a chemical called adenosine that helps support your sleep drive. Caffeine blocks the adenosine actions and counteracts sleepiness.

Amygdala: It's an almond-shaped structure in your brain that becomes active during the REM sleep stage and helps processing emotions.

1.2) Sleep Stages

Following are the two basic sleep types:

- REM (rapid eye movement) sleep
- Non-REM sleep (which has three different stages).

Each sleep type is linked to a particular neuronal activity and brain wave. During your sleep, you cycle through all the REM and non-REM sleep stages several times.

1.2.1) REM sleep

You reach this stage typically in about ninety minutes after falling asleep. During REM sleep, your eyes move behind closed eyelids rapidly from side to side and most of your dreaming occurs in this stage. Some dreaming also occurs during non-REM sleep. Your breathing turns irregular and faster, and your blood pressure and heart rate increase to near waking levels. The muscles of your arms and legs become paralyzed temporarily so that you don't act out your dreams. Both REM and non-REM sleep is necessary for memory consolidation.

1.2.2) Non-REM sleep

Non-REM sleep has three different stages:

- **Non-REM Sleep Stage 1:** This stage is very light sleep that comprises about 5% of your sleep time. You can easily wake up from this stage. It lasts for a short period (a few minutes). During stage 1, your eye movements, breathing, and heartbeat slow down, and your muscles relax with infrequent twitches. Even your brain waves start to slow from its daytime alertness patterns.

- **Non-REM Sleep Stage 2:** This stage is also light sleep but it should comprise about 45 to 55% of your sleep time. It's a light sleep before entering deeper sleep when your breathing, heartbeat, and muscles relax even more. Your eye movements stop, and your body temperature dips. Although the brain wave slows, there're short bursts of electrical activity.

- **Non-REM Sleep Stage 3:** This stage is of deep sleep and it should comprise about 20% of your sleep time so that you feel refreshed in the morning. At this stage, your breathing, heartbeat, and brain waves slow down to their lowest levels. The muscles stay relaxed and it could be difficult to wake you up.

1.3) How many hours do you need to sleep?

As you age, your sleep patterns and need for sleep changes. However, your need for sleep varies considerably across the same age individuals. There is no fixed number of sleep hours, which works for every individual of the same age.

Babies can sleep up to 16–18 hours per day that is essential for their body growth and brain development. Toddlers, school-age kids, and teenagers need about 9½ hours of sleep per day. Adults typically require 7-8 hours of sleep per day.

As you age, especially after 60, your sleep may get lighter and shorter. Your sleep may also be disrupted by multiple awakenings. Certain medications taken by elderly people may also interfere with their sleep.

Furthermore, in today's time, people are getting less sleep owing to a number of factors such as stress, anxiety, long working hours, overindulgence in round-the-clock entertainment, excess LED screen exposure, etc.

You might think you can make up for the missed sleep hours during the weekend. However, depending on how sleep-deprived you are, long weekend slumbers may not be sufficient.

During sleep, your body goes through a series of changes that facilitate sleep, which is essential for your overall health. Sleep lets your body and brain to slow down and take part in the recovery processes, which, in turn, result in better mental and physical performance the next day and in the long run.

Lack of sleep can short-circuit these fundamental processes, which can adversely affect your thinking patterns, focus, mood, and energy levels. Therefore, getting adequate sleep you need is crucial.

The way your body and brain functions during sleep and the different stages of sleep shows the complexity of sleep and its significance for your overall well-being.

1.4) How your body and brain function during sleep?

During your sleep, nearly every part of your body goes through notable changes. According to a **study done by NCBI[3]**, during your sleep, thousands of neurons inside your brain transmits signals all over your body to switch from waking to a sleeping state.

The study further revealed that sleep not only reinforces your immune and cardiovascular systems but also helps regulate metabolism. Following are some notable changes in your core bodily functions that occur during sleep:

- **Heart Rate:** During Stage 1 sleep, the heart rate starts to slow down, and during Stage 3, it reaches its slowest pace. On the contrary, the heart rate speeds up during REM sleep to almost the same rate when you're awake.
- **Breathing:** During non-REM sleep, breathing slows and reaches its lowest rates during stage 3 sleep. But, during REM sleep, breathing becomes faster and could be irregular.
- **Muscle Tone:** A **study conducted by NCBI[4]** revealed that during each stage of non-REM sleep, the total energy expenditure of your body drops that results in muscle relaxation. On the contrary, most muscles remain in a paralyzed condition called atonia during the REM stage to prevent you from responding to your dreams. Eye muscles and the respiratory system remain active. The eyes

keep moving behind closed eyelids, which inspired the name REM (Rapid Eye Movement) sleep.

- **Brain Activity:** Brain waves slow down significantly during the non-REM stage 1 sleep. But, during non-REM Stage 2 and Stage 3, there are frequent rapid bursts of brain activity. Brain activity speeds up during REM sleep and clearly becomes different types of brain waves. Since brain activity gets heightened during REM sleep, this stage is most connected to vivid dreaming. According to **research done by Harvard**[5] medical school, REM sleep may enable vital cognitive abilities such as memory consolidation. Although non-REM sleep has reduced brain activity, it may also play a significant role in proper brain functioning.
- **Hormone Levels: An NCBI study**[6] suggests that your circadian rhythm plays a significant role in regulating the production of the following hormones:

  1. **Melatonin:** It helps promote sleep.
  2. **Cortisol:** It's a part of the stress response system in your body.
  3. **Growth hormone:** It supports metabolism as well as muscle and bone development.

During different stages of sleep, the levels of hormones may vary, and the quality of sleep can affect hormone production when you're awake during the daytime.

- **Dreaming:** During REM sleep, dreaming is believed to be most intense and prevalent. But, **an NCBI study**[7] suggests that dreaming can occur during any sleep stage. Another **NCBI study**[8] suggests that dreams that occur during REM and non-REM sleep tends to show distinct patterns. REM dreams are often more bizarre, immersive, or imaginary.

Sleep disorders can have a negative impact on your overall well-being.

For example, disrupted breathing (sleep apnea) or restless leg syndrome can result in frequent awakenings that disrupt your normal sleep cycle.

As a result, you may not get the restorative benefits of quality sleep. Sleep disorders can severely disrupt your circadian rhythm (sleep-wake cycle) that can result in abnormal sleeping habits or insufficient sleep.

1.5) Insomnia

If you're finding it hard to fall asleep, you're most likely suffering from insomnia. People with insomnia get insufficient sleep, so they may develop abnormal sleeping habits. To get proper rest, you need to progress through all the sleep stages. If you don't sleep well, it may result in daytime sleepiness that can have negative effects on your health, mood, and thinking.

Insomnia or sleep deprivation can severely disrupt the balance of your sleep architecture. An NCBI study revealed that people with insomnia often experience a **REM sleep rebound**[9]. It means they tend to spend an inconsistent amount of time in the REM sleep stage. This can result in excess brain activity that can leave you with irritable feelings. This can worsen any mental health problems like depression and anxiety.

1.6) Hypersomnia

Hypersomnia or excess sleep is a condition when you sleep too much. If you suffer from hypersomnia, you'll often experience abnormal daytime sleepiness and you may find it difficult to remain awake when you need to.

An NCBI research suggests that hypersomnia condition is related to **changes in sleep architecture**[10], for example, reduced deep sleep and increased non-REM sleep that can impact the overall sleep quality.

1.7) Quality Sleep for Spiritual Well-being

A good night's sleep can also be achieved by embracing your spiritual side. You need to turn off your mind and try to get more in tune with nature and spirituality to attain the benefits of quality sleep.

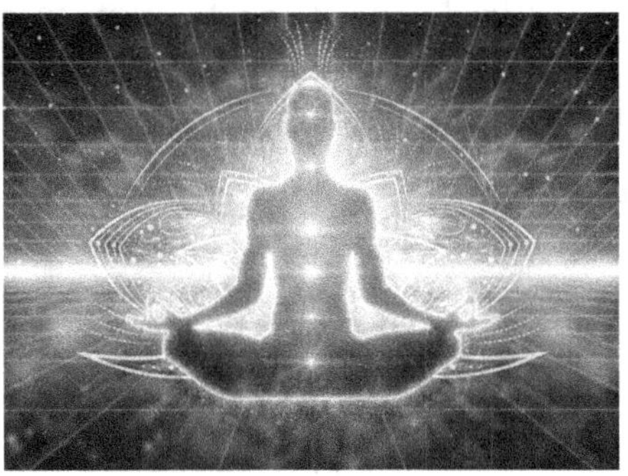

You can achieve inner peace by embracing spirituality. Everything around us is connected to the concept of spirituality. We have a meaningful existence in the world around us and we are an important part of it. There is a force or power that is superior to us.

Various scientific studies suggest that following a spiritual path is the sure-shot way to happiness. You won't suffer from anxiety and depression when you get in touch with your spiritual side. This is also applicable to how well you sleep at night. If you remain stressed out all the time, most likely you won't sleep well.

When you embrace your spirituality, both your physical and mental health improves. When you put energy into improving one aspect of yourself, the other aspects benefit. This is how a holistic approach works.

Try to meditate in the evening for better sleep. Practicing meditation will have a calming effect on your brain cells and nerves after a stressful day. It'll also help lower your blood pressure. Meditation can help your mind attain more focus that'll help you reflect and organize your thoughts in a more positive manner. Your organized mind will allow you to stay more relaxed at the end of the day.

A Harvard University study[11] in 2015 revealed that people sleep better post-meditation. Meditation can effectively make you feel calm and relaxed when you need it most. Spirituality and meditation go hand -in-hand. The more you practice meditation, the more you'll consider yourself an important part of the world around you.

The circadian rhythm of your body is associated with the hours of sunlight. So, you need to follow the seasons. Since the days are longer during summers, it's natural to get-up early and go to sleep slightly late in the evening. But during winters, the days get shorter. So, to wake-up feeling refreshed, you may feel the need for an extra hour of night's sleep during winters.

The regrets of the day can cause a lot of stress. There may be numerous things in your mind that can disrupt your peaceful sleep. You may have sleep troubles because you're re-living conversations that you might have had during the day. Maybe you're thinking of things you wish you wouldn't have said or said.

To let go of any regrets, visualize them before going to bed. Your regrets aren't worth dwelling on. You need to learn from your past mistakes, let them go, and begin the next day with a refreshed energy after a good night's sleep. You need to differentiate between the things you can change and the things you can't. You can't change your past mistakes.

It's important to go to bed in the right frame of mind. While you try to fall asleep, think about the places that you wish to visit or feel most connected to. For example, beach, river, ocean, or forest. To help slow your heart rate and focus your breathing, you can listen to the sounds of nature.

Your brain activity changes when you fall asleep and it's a gradual process. To help your brain and body fall asleep quickly, you can visualize your thoughts. Imagine yourself entering a warm sea. Slowly relax each part of your body, as you move in deeper, from your feet upwards. Feel them getting heavier and sinking into the bed.

To get a good night's sleep, you need to limit your nighttime distractions. Before going to bed, use meditation or visualization to focus on your inner thoughts and ward off mental stresses to achieve all the benefits of a good night's sleep.

In the next chapter, we'll discuss how to TRAIN YOUR MIND to sleep better.

Do We Need To Train Ourselves To Sleep Better?

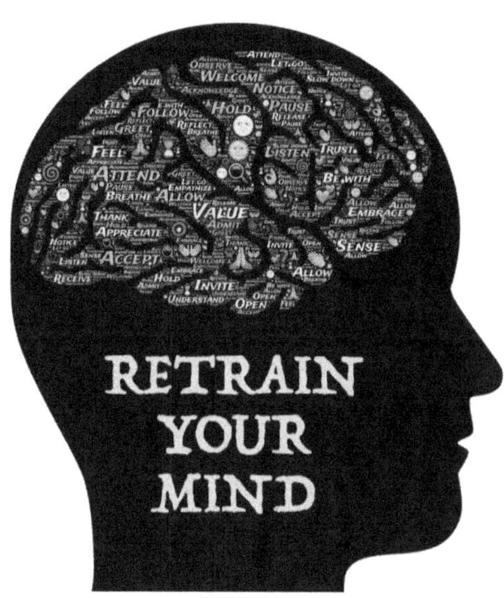

Let's assume you have sleep troubles but you are firm to get your full 7-8 hours sleep and every night you make efforts to achieve this goal. You go to sleep at the exact same time, no matter whether you're tired or not.

But, all night long you're not able to sleep. You keep tossing and turning. You yell at your mind to calm down. You gaze at the alarm clock and make deals with yourself like "If I fall asleep at this moment, I'll still get 3 hours!" After hours of screaming at your loud brain, at last, you close your eyes and get 30 minutes of sleep, and the alarm goes off!

There could be a large mental aspect that prevents you from getting quality sleep. This mental aspect may become evident as a racing mind that wakes you up several times in the night for no real reason and prevents you from falling asleep.

The truth is you've trained your brain to relate your sleep with feelings of anxiety, stress, and constant worry. This can worsen during high-stress times like

COVID-19.

When you don't get enough sleep, your focus and attention abilities decline. You become less attentive; your reaction time extends, and you don't react well to environmental signals. This means you lose the ability to acquire new information or respond to dangerous circumstances, for example, when you're driving a car.

However, you can definitely un-train your mind and then retrain it to relate your sleep with a calm and serene mind to achieve a good night's sleep.

There are multiple techniques that you can use to train your mind to sleep faster, better, and deeper. Following are some of the proven solid techniques backed by numerous scientific studies:

2.1) CBT (Cognitive Behavioral Therapy)

CBT is primarily based on stoic philosophy. This therapy involves using your brain to critically think about your thinking patterns, and then actively start thinking in a different way.

CBT is an effective therapy because your brain has the ability to recognize and create patterns. Sleep is just another pattern that can be influenced by your mind.

This therapy addresses your negative behavior and thinking patterns, which contribute to sleep disorders such as insomnia. CBT involves the following main components:

Cognitive therapy: This teaches you to identify and transform negative thoughts and beliefs, which contribute to your sleep troubles.

Behavioral therapy: This teaches you the ways to steer clear of behaviors that disrupt your sleep at night and switch them with good sleep habits.

In a **placebo-controlled clinical trial**[12], CBT was tested on 78 older adult participants along with other traditional pharmacological tests to treat their insomnia. The study revealed that CBT alone could significantly reduce insomnia by as much as 55 percent.

CBT when combined with other traditional pharmaceuticals could boost the effectiveness by as much as 63 percent.

The clinical trial further revealed that the participants treated with CBT continued to sleep better. However, those participants who only took traditional pharmaceuticals lost sleep benefits once they stopped taking the medications.

2.2) Hypnosis & Hypnotherapy

Derived from the Greek word "Hypnos", hypnosis as a therapeutic tool has been utilized for thousands of years. But, it has been only recently understood from a scientific perspective.

Contrary to a popular misconception, modern-day hypnosis won't leave you unconscious. A hypnotherapist uses hypnosis to bring about a hypnotic trance, a self-directed altered state, which leaves you more receptive to beneficial instructions.

As a certified hypnotherapist and mind coach, I have often encountered several misconceptions of hypnosis like:

It's magical: In truth, hypnosis is a natural and enhanced state of learning. There is nothing magical about it, although the effects can seem magic on occasion.

You're asleep when experiencing hypnosis: In truth, you typically remain very relaxed when experiencing hypnosis, but not asleep. You remain alert but in a calm state.

It's dangerous: Since hypnosis is a completely natural state, it can't be dangerous. However, it's a powerful therapy and it should be treated with respect. Hypnosis should only be administered by a trained professional such as www.basingstokehypnotherapy4you.com

You'll lose control in Hypnosis: In truth, your mind remains in control in a state of hypnosis. You'll not do or say anything against your wish. This mistaken belief is due to the stage hypnosis that uses the natural suggestibility of extremely susceptible people to perform funny things, which they happily do. But, stage hypnotists always pick their subjects quite carefully. They test suggestible people because they know that such subjects will be good for entertainment purposes. The use of hypnosis within hypnotherapy is entirely different from stage hypnosis.

Not everyone can be hypnotized: In truth, everyone can be hypnotized and can achieve a deep trance state. When in hypnosis, each individual experiences different things, but it's only the very young and the elderly who may find it difficult to achieve a heightened state of consciousness since their level of focus is usually lower. As a pre-requisite of hypnosis is the ability to concentrate and imagine.

Someone else controls you in hypnosis: In truth, no one can force you into hypnosis. You'll always be able to control your mind. Your professional www.basingstokehypnotherapy4you.com facilitates the process and helps to produce the therapeutic change you desire.

2.2.1) Hypnosis

Hypnosis could be described as an enhanced state of learning or an altered state of consciousness that arises as a result of changes in your brain. Although such changes can also naturally happen in certain circumstances, in hypnosis, a hypnotherapist induces this state by using specific techniques.

Here, your attention stays narrowed and focused. Hypnosis creates an environment where your brain processes information differently, allowing you to access further areas of your brain.

In a hypnotic state, you'll be able to learn new beliefs and new habits much faster. Modern-day hypnosis is interlinked with the latest and ever-evolving practical neuroscience that keeps exploring how the human brain functions.

Although hypnosis and sleep have countless similarities, they are not at all similar. During hypnosis, your body will feel extremely relaxed and you'll remain still. You'll feel as if your body has gone to sleep. In reality, you stay awake. The unconscious part of your brain becomes more active and the conscious part of your brain is turned off.

Multiple scientific studies have shown that hypnotic relaxation techniques can help improve sleep. An **NCBI study was conducted on teens**[13] for the treatment of insomnia. In the study, hypnosis was used together with CBT and progressive muscle relaxation to improve the quality of sleep in the participants.

2.2.2) Hypnotherapy

Hypnotherapy is an approach that utilizes the state of hypnosis as its key therapeutic tool. It's a tried and tested technique that utilizes the power of the mind to help improve your mental and physical well-being.

Hypnosis results in significant changes in thinking patterns. The brain processes information differently during the state of hypnosis. These changes can be used to produce therapeutic change.

Hypnosis lets you sidestep the limitation of your conscious mind and thoughts. It improves your creativity and imaginative ability by processing information in a different way.

A qualified hypnotherapist utilizes such abilities to help address your problems productively. He/she can help you access your subconscious mind under a state of hypnosis to help you achieve your goals through improved thought processes.

2.2.3) How do you feel under hypnosis?

Although you might feel some magical effects of hypnosis, there is nothing magical about it. Every hypnosis experience is unique but most people have experienced some common aspects.

In hypnosis, you enter a trance state or an altered state of consciousness. This state is similar to feeling so engrossed in a task such as playing chess or reading a book that you are totally unaware of what's happening around you and the passing time as if you are in a zone. This is similar to a trance state or an altered state of consciousness.

Simply put, the state of hypnosis is similar to the experience you get moments before drifting off to sleep. Your mind wanders and feels calm and relaxed. Your body feels asleep, but you're mentally aware. You experience deep relaxation paired with an altered state of consciousness. You may also feel detached from the outside world, for example, traffic outside would be clearly audible to you but it may sound distant or irrelevant.

In the state of hypnosis, you may often experience some sensation in your body specifically in the limbs. You may also experience a sense of floating, feeling light, or not being aware of your body.

In hypnosis, you may also experience time distortion. You

may feel that you've been in a trance for just a few moments when, in reality, thirty minutes have passed. Quite the opposite, you may feel relaxed for half an hour, but, in reality, merely a few minutes have passed.

2.2.4) Hypnosis and Your Brain

If you have the basic knowledge of how the brain functions in relation to hypnosis, you'll understand how to utilize it as a therapeutic tool. The state of hypnosis is created by changes in the brain, which allows the processing of information differently. It is the reprocessing that results in therapeutic change.

The changes in your brain occur as a result of changes in your autonomic nervous system. Following are the two main parts of your autonomic nervous system:

Sympathetic nervous system: It is dominant when you feel threatened, stressed, or aroused. It's also called the "fight or flight" mode. As your body prepares for action, your heart races fast, your blood pressure rises, and you sweat a lot.

Parasympathetic nervous system: It is dominant when your body feels calm and relaxed. As your body reaches a relaxed state, your breathing slows, your heart slows, and all the bodily functions slow.

In hypnosis, the altered state of consciousness is initiated when the autonomic nervous system is switched to the parasympathetic dominance state.

2.3) Fundamentals of Human Brain

Your brain primarily controls your whole body and mind. Although the evolution of the human brain has spanned over millions of years, the basic human brain remains similar to the brain of the first evolved human.

Several traits and features of the human brain are in common with other mammals. The only difference is that the human brain is more conscious and evolved. But, the unconscious part of your brain holds more importance in some ways. As a human, you tend to focus more on your conscious abilities and since you possess the ability to communicate with language and words, you tend to over-rely on your conscious abilities.

Yet, most of the information processing takes place in the unconscious part of your brain. Your brain processes the information from the internal bodily states and the external world. The data travels back and forth between your brain and the rest of your body through nerve impulses. Your brain utilizes this process to regulate conscious and unconscious body processes. A hypnotic state develops through these processes.

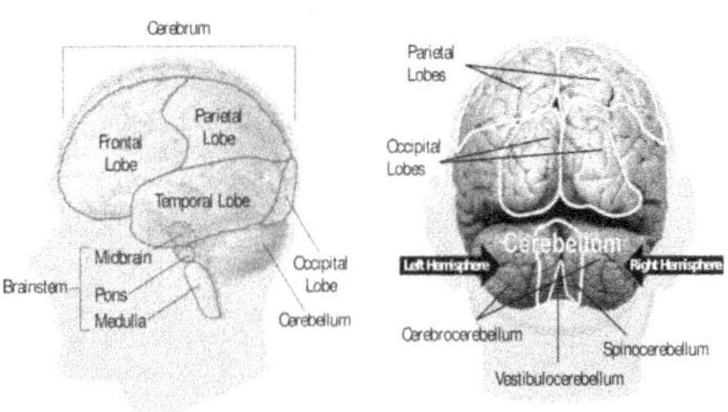

2.3.1) Cerebral Cortex

It's the largest part of the human brain that covers nearly two–thirds of the entire brain mass. The cerebral cortex is considered the most recent structure in the evolution of the human brain.

The cerebral cortex shapes your brain's outer layer and comprises a heavily-folded grey surface. Its key responsibility is producing and understanding language, and the conscious awareness of behaviors and thoughts.

The frontal lobe, the cortex's front part, is explicitly involved in the conscious awareness in skill movements, emotional thoughts, and decision making. Behind the frontal lobe lies the parietal lobe that recognizes and interprets sensations such as pain, temperature, and touch.

At the rear of your brain is the occipital lobe that is responsible for visual images. On either side of the cortex lie the temporal lobes that are responsible for hearing and certain cognitive processing. Most of the processing in the cerebral cortex remains unconscious. However, conscious awareness starts from your brain's outer layer. In the state of hypnosis, this conscious part of your brain becomes less active.

The cortex is divided into two equal halves know as hemispheres, which are connected together. The hemispheres communicate with each other via the corpus callosum, which is a huge bundle of nerve fibers.

In hypnosis, brain activity changes between the hemispheres. Heightened activity between the hemispheres brings about some hypnotic phenomena, for example, time perception distortion, enhanced visual imagery, and surreal thoughts.

2.3.2) Limbic System

The limbic system is located deep inside your brain on top of your brain stem and underneath your cerebral cortex. It administers the rest of your brain and body.

The limbic system processes the information before you are even aware of it, so its processes are unconscious. It controls the level of brain activity in your cortex. The limbic region sends signals to the conscious parts of your brain and regulates memory, learning, emotions, and attention.

In hypnosis, changes in the limbic system help produce an altered state of consciousness. These changes in the limbic system are also vital to the therapeutic benefits associated with hypnosis.

2.3.3) Cerebellum and Brain stem

The prime responsibility of the cerebellum and the brain stem is to monitor nearly all the basic functioning of your body. Both are quite old in terms of evolution. They help regulate numerous life-support mechanisms, for example, your blood pressure, basic body movements, heart rate, breathing, and digestion.

Your brain stem is crucial for maintaining consciousness. In hypnosis, it plays a critical role in the altered state of consciousness. All information transmitted from your brain to the body, and vice versa, ought to pass through the brain stem. All sensory experiences, such as touch, temperature, and pain, are communicated via the brain stem. During hypnosis, these experiences are often changed, which indicates an altered brain stem activity.

Your cerebellum contains more brain cells (neurons) than all the remaining parts of your brain put together. Earlier the prime role of the cerebellum was considered to be the co-ordination of body movements. But, in the last two decades, new evidence emerged, which revealed that the cerebellum is also responsible for memory, attention, mental imagery, and language.

Your cerebellum doesn't follow the two-way communication system unlike other areas of your brain. It typically sends out more signals to your brain than it receives from the brain. In hypnosis, changes in the cerebellum can most likely mediate numerous changes in conscious awareness.

2.4) How your brain functions as a whole?

Your cerebellum and the brain stem are considered as the foundations. Although they may not be sufficient for human existence, they are surely essential for human life. Your brain's limbic region functions as a control center of your body and brain. The limbic system is unconscious and controls the activity of the cortex region.

Your cortex allows you to be conscious of your human experiences. In hypnosis, the limbic region is the most important part for the following two reasons:

The changes in the limbic system produce a hypnotic experience.

These changes bring about the therapeutic benefits of hypnosis.

Your limbic system includes several important structures like the thalamus, hypothalamus, hippocampus, amygdale, cingulate gyrus, nucleus accumbens, and insula.

All these structures not only communicate with each other, but also with other extensive areas of your brain such as the cortex and the brain stem, and the rest of your body.

2.5) Hypnosis and Brain Activity

In hypnosis, certain changes occur in your brain's electrical activity, which is mediated by a structure in your limbic system called the cingulate gyrus. Such changes in the electrical activity of your brain can be measured by a technique called electroencephalography (EEG).

In the EEG test, electrodes are placed on your scalp to record the electrical activity level in your brain. Your brain is typically in an alert state when you're awake, or at work, or talking to friends. These are reflected in short and spiky BETA brain waves, which show a lot of activities going on.

In contrast, your brain shows slower and gentler ALPHA brain waves, when you feel more relaxed, for example, while listening to music or watching television.

When you're asleep, your brain reaches an even more relaxed state and exhibits DELTA brain waves that are much slower, aside from the REM (Rapid Eye Movement) sleep stage when your brain activity increases temporarily.

During hypnosis, your brain

attains a different form that is neither asleep nor awake but is both relaxed and active. In hypnosis, your brain produces THETA brain waves. This is the main hypnosis.

2.6) How hypnosis make your brain function at a different rate?

In hypnosis, various techniques are used to produce the altered state of consciousness through numerous mechanisms. One such mechanism involves changes in your autonomic nervous system.

We have already discussed in section 2.2.4 (Hypnosis and Your Brain) of this chapter about how in hypnosis the altered state of consciousness is initiated when the autonomic nervous system is switched to the parasympathetic dominance state.

Many hypnosis techniques support parasympathetic dominance as this helps create a state where your brain easily produces ALPHA and THETA brain waves that reflect a deep calm state.

The pituitary gland is a tiny structure deep inside your brain that controls the secretion of hormones. This gland receives chemical messages from the hypothalamus of your brain. These messages then move down the body to the top of your kidneys where your adrenal glands are located.

The adrenal glands, in turn, control the stress hormone levels in your body that further activates your sympathetic nervous system that regulates your "fight or flight" mode.

2.7) What's the role of the HPA axis in hypnosis?

In hypnosis, you enter into an altered state of consciousness and become more relaxed. This relaxed state sends signals to your HPA axis that there's no imminent danger and it is safe for your body and mind to switch to a parasympathetic dominance state.

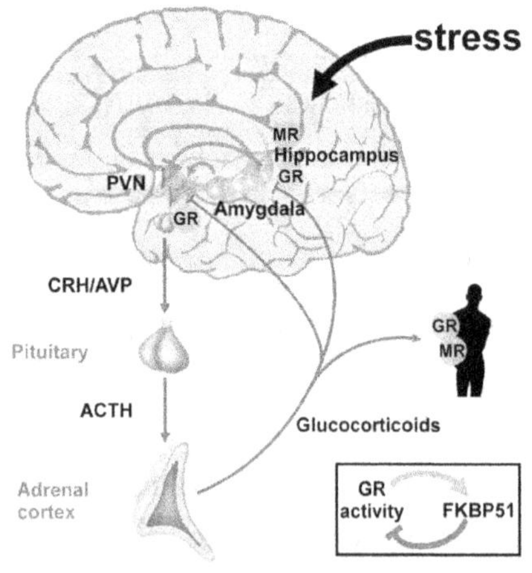

Courtesy: Wikimedia Commons

This leads to even deeper levels of physical and mental relaxation, which is similar to deep sleep. But, in reality, you still remain awake and have conscious awareness.

The HPA (hypothalamic-pituitary-adrenal) explains the interaction between the pituitary gland, hypothalamus, and adrenal glands. The main function of the HPA axis involves the reaction of your body to stress.

When your body and mind experience something stressful, your sympathetic nervous system mediates the initial response to the stress. This response happens almost instantly and leads to the secretion of hormones such as epinephrine and norepinephrine. Both hormones work to carry out changes if you feel frightened or stressed out such as increased perspiration and heart rate.

The HPA axis gets stimulated nearly 10 seconds later. The hypothalamus secretes CRH (corticotropin-releasing hormone) into your bloodstream in response to the signals like increased norepinephrine levels. CRH itself elevates the activity of the sympathetic nervous system that perpetuates the effects such as increased heart rate.

Furthermore, CRH also instructs your pituitary gland to secrete a hormone called ACTH (adrenocorticotropic hormone). After ACTH is released into your bloodstream by the pituitary gland, it travels down to the outer layer of your adrenal glands called the adrenal cortex.

Once ACTH reaches the adrenal cortex, it binds to the receptors on the cortex's surface that further leads to a series of intracellular actions, which result in the adrenal glands secreting glucocorticoids such as the hormone cortisol.

Hormone cortisol has numerous effects on your body, which are believed to be carried out with the purpose of helping your body deal with a number of stressors. For instance, cortisol helps increase cardiac output and blood pressure to supply more blood to your skeletal muscles if the stressor involves some type of physical effort. Cortisol also helps increase glucose levels in your blood. Glucose provides your body cells with crucial energy to help cope with the stressor.

In addition, the cortisol hormone acts, at the time when your body experiences a serious stressor, to slow down those processes that are of lesser importance at that time. For instance, reproductive activity gets reduced.

From the perspective of your body, the bodily activities that don't let you cope with the stressor at hand ought to be ignored until the severe stress ends. For example, when dealing with an acute stressor, you should not become preoccupied with sex. You should rather consider it to be more of a leisure activity.

Although proper HPA axis functioning is necessary for dealing with stress, its excess stimulation can result in psychiatric and physical problems. An **NCBI study**[14] suggests that increased cortisol levels may suppress immune system response in people making them more vulnerable to infection.

Another **NCBI study**[15] suggests that repeated HPA axis activation may result in cardiovascular disease, obesity, and type-2 diabetes. A different **NCBI study**[16] suggests that cortisol may have harmful effects on cognition and memory. Another **NCBI study**[17] suggests that increased cortisol levels are associated with mood disorders such as depression.

Furthermore, your early life experiences can affect your HPA axis's baseline activity. An **NCBI research**[18] revealed that early-life trauma may result in an over-reactive HPA axis. Another **NCBI research**[19] revealed that an over-reactive HPA axis can lead to elevated anxiety levels and possible metabolic effects such as excess insulin resistance and fat deposition.

Therefore, your HPA axis needs to function properly to help you to deal effectively with stressors. But, the beneficial role of your HPA axis can be disrupted by repeated stress.

Your HPA axis represents an important area to explore and a possible target for therapeutic medicines due to its significant role in a strong response to stress and disease.

2.8) Reticular Activating System (RAS)

During sleep, you basically experience three sleep and arousal states – awake, asleep (slow-wave sleep or resting), and dreaming (REM sleep, active, or paradoxical). The RAS controls and regulates these sleep and waking states, as well as your 'fight-or-flight' modes.

The RAS is a network of neurons that spans a wide portion of your brainstem. Most of these neurons are in the reticular formation and the network performs the arousal and alerting functions.

The RAS activities are modulated by complex interactions between numerous neurotransmitters where both adrenergic and cholinergic neurotransmitters play key roles.

The ascending RAS projects to the thalami's intralaminar nuclei that projects in a diffuse manner to the cerebral cortex. The ascending RAS projections elevate the attentive state of the cerebral cortex and enable conscious awareness of sensory stimuli. In addition, the combined role of your brainstem reticular formation is to control and regulate your muscle reflexes, autonomic function, and mood.

The RAS regulates your fight-or-flight modes, so you may feel that responses to sudden alerting stimuli are abnormal. For example, an overactive RAS results in disorders such as PTSD (posttraumatic stress disorder). This means that such stimuli may produce overstressed responses such as hyperactive reflexes or exaggerated shock reactions.

Also, RAS is known for its rapid habituation (decrease in response) to recurring stimuli. It lacks responsiveness to rapidly recurring stimuli. For example, in the case of PTSD disorder, there could be a sensory gating deficit or decrease in habituation.

Waking and sleep are controlled by the RAS to regulate your sleep patterns. The upregulation of the RAS may lead to difficulty in getting and maintaining sleep, which can result in insomnia, decreased slow-wave sleep, irregular sleep, and increased REM sleep drive characterized by frequent nightmares and repeated awakenings.

2.9) How your mind affects your body?

According to the past western philosophy, the mind and body were considered as separate entities, and it was assumed that thoughts had no effect on the body. However, with the rapid development of science, it was profoundly established that the mind, emotions, beliefs, and thoughts can affect the human body. There is a neurological consequence behind every thought. Thoughts affect your brain, which, in turn, can affect your whole body.

2.10) Conscious and unconscious processing

During hypnosis, the brain changes allow you to access those regions of your brain that typically remain inaccessible and unconscious. In truth, the conscious part of your brain that allows you to be conscious is just the tip of the iceberg.

The unconscious part of your brain always works behind the scenes. For example, your brain doesn't consciously register much of what you hear and see. That information is processed unconsciously. Subsequently, some of that processed information attains conscious awareness.

2.11) Conscious Mind and Subconscious Mind

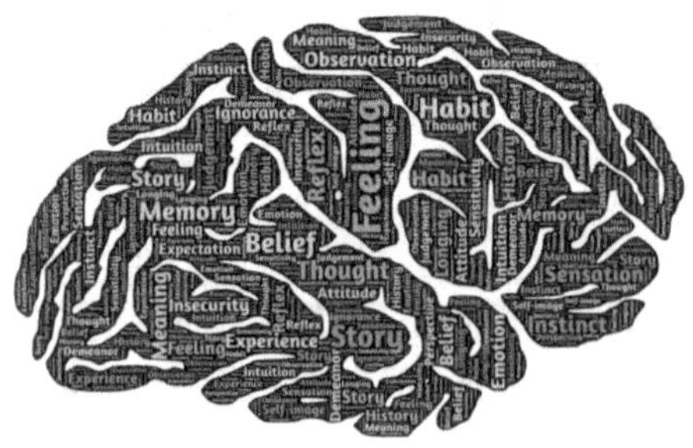

As a certified hypnotherapist, I often receive hundreds of queries about how hypnosis actually works. Let me explain to you why I believe it is one of the most powerful tools for change.

Your first step is to understand the concept of – "One Brain Two Minds". What does it mean? We all have one brain, but we possess two minds – CONSCIOUS MIND and SUBCONSCIOUS MIND.

To understand hypnosis, it is essential to understand how the CONSCIOUS MIND and SUBCONSCIOUS MIND function. Each mind has different abilities, functions, and capacities.

2.11.1) Conscious Mind

CONSCIOUS mind represents your daily normal state of awareness. However, the CONSCIOUS mind is rather limited. It carries out some critical functions. For example, it's really good at planning things; setting up goals; and breaking things down into steps to make sure you achieve those goals. In the absence of a CONSCIOUS mind, you wouldn't be able to achieve your goals, since you can't plan effectively.

The best attribute of your CONSCIOUS mind is that it lets you attain self-awareness. Without CONSCIOUS mind, you won't be able to realize the beauty of the scenery. You won't be falling in love. You won't be appreciating the task you've done and feel proud of your accomplishments. Your CONSCIOUS mind allows you to appreciate all the good things in your life. It lets you decide what more you want from your life.

Most importantly, your CONSCIOUS mind is the place where logic and reasoning rests, which is a very valuable skill.

2.11.2) Subconscious Mind

Your SUBCONSCIOUS mind is the place where your record and act in response to habits. It's the place where your memories, wisdom, intuitions, learning, insights, and happy and unpleasant experiences are stored. Besides, it's your connection with Higher Intelligence.

A fair comparison between your CONSCIOUS and SUBCONSCIOUS mind is to visualize a captain, his crew, and his ship. Consider your CONSCIOUS mind as the captain, and the crew and ship as your SUBCONSCIOUS mind. The captain is responsible to set the direction and instruct the crew on what to do.

Therefore, the key difference between your CONSCIOUS and SUBCONSCIOUS mind is that one furnishes directions and the other follows the directions.

Right from the moment you wake up, to the moment you go to sleep, you mostly function from your SUBCONSCIOUS mind.

2.11.3) Critical Faculty

The Critical Faculty is the division between your SUBCONSCIOUS and CONSCIOUS mind. The Faculty takes the thoughts of your CONSCIOUS mind and seeks approval from your SUBCONSCIOUS mind to deliver the information along. Sometimes your SUBCONSCIOUS mind allows the information to be delivered and sometimes it disallows.

It's a general belief that humans develop this Critical Faculty at the age of six. Through the first 6 years of human life, the prenatal and neonatal brains function mainly in Delta and Theta EEG frequencies. This brain activity level is also considered as the state of hypnosis.

In this state of hypnosis, kids don't need to be actively coached into particular beliefs. They develop their core belief system just by interacting and observing their parents, peers, siblings, television, teachers, and religion.

Kids learn things really quickly up to the age of six. You can observe how quickly kids can pick up new information. The reason behind this is their Critical Faculty is not yet developed.

As kids grow, they start to learn to understand the difference between right and wrong, and the importance of exercising caution. As a result, their Critical Faculty gradually turns more sharp and developed.

After the development of the Critical Faculty, it brings about a new set of problems. For example, if you're a smoker, your Conscious Mind will tell you to quit smoking. The Critical Faculty will seek approval from your SUBCONSCIOUS mind if that thought is allowed to enter.

Your SUBCONSCIOUS mind governs your habits including smoking. Although your mind knows that smoking is injurious to health, your SUBCONSCIOUS mind always resists changes and adopt the path of least resistance. As a result, your SUBCONSCIOUS mind will not allow that thought to enter.

The SUBCONSCIOUS mind hates changes and prefers to operate on the principle of minimal effort. It prefers routine and favors things the way they are. So, it may try to make excuses to validate the decision to keep smoking like "Smoking helps reduce stress", and most likely it'll reject the 'quit smoking' message.

However, once you're able to substitute these hidden SUBCONSCIOUS blocks and beliefs, nothing will stop you from changing any habit or any aspect of your life. You'll certainly become a non-smoker. All roadblocks will disappear.

The Critical Faculty is also known as the Gatekeeper. As the name implies, it controls or limits, in a manipulative way, what you allow inside from the outer world.

The gatekeeper's function is quite simple — to keep things the same. Its main objective is to snub information that doesn't match with the likings of your Subconscious mind to make your life easier.

Some very powerful tools that the Gatekeeper has at its disposal include emotions such as fear, worry, anger, and doubt. These tools are psychological defense mechanisms, which automatically decline new information.

The Gatekeeper can be very useful to thwart off stupid information. But, it'll also stop you from making new decisions. It can also very harmful when it keeps you stuck with a bad habit or belief, which you don't want anymore.

2.12) Reality of Willpower

You might try to change your beliefs and habits by using your willpower. You'll say to yourself everyday "I WILL stop smoking", "I WILL be confident", "I WILL lose weight", or "I WILL become successful", etc.

However, the truth is – there no such thing as Willpower! It doesn't exist!

You do not lack willpower or have surplus willpower. In reality, when you use the term "willpower", your Conscious mind is trying to override your Subconscious mind. Simply put, your Conscious mind can always override your SUBCONSCIOUS mind. For instance, if you consciously make a decision to not smoke, most likely you won't smoke, but only for a while. The moment you feel stressed or distracted, your SUBCONSCIOUS mind will tell you to smoke, and you'll again end up smoking.

When you use the term willpower to consciously change your habits or beliefs, your commitment might work for a short time. But, as soon as you feel stressed or lose your focus, your SUBCONSCIOUS mind takes over, and you end up the way you were before you tried to make the change.

2.13) How to persuade your mind to make changes?

Firstly, you need to understand that you don't lack the will to make changes. You are simply having difficulties making ones. The real reason you're unable to make the essential changes is you're employing the wrong part of your mind to bring about those changes. You're putting all your focus in the wrong place.

You need to change your automatic programming or the SUBCONSCIOUS Blueprint, or else you'll get the same outcomes again and again no matter how hard you try.

Hypnosis is one of the fastest ways to change your SUBCONSCIOUS Blueprint. Hypnosis bypasses the Gatekeeper (the Critical Faculty) letting you rewrite your SUBCONSCIOUS Blueprint. That's how it helps you achieve everything you want from life without any struggles or efforts.

When it comes to manifesting your intentions, an important thing to understand is that your Subconscious mind doesn't change immediately or conduct instant action.

You need to allow your SUBCONSCIOUS to take its time to make the changes. The existing Blueprint inside your mind took time to set. Likewise, it'll take some time for that blueprint to change.

A professional hypnotherapist can help you change your SUBCONSCIOUS Blueprint a lot quicker using hypnosis. In hypnosis, your SUBCONSCIOUS will be allowed to perform its chores and bring you whatever you desire.

Hypnosis is a potent tool for bringing change including having a good night's sleep. Your professional www.basingstoke hypnotherapy4you.com facilitates the process and helps to produce the therapeutic change you desire.

Log on to **https:// www.basingstokehypnotherapy 4you.com/book-purchase- audios** to download HYPNOTIC AUDIOS your access password is in the reference section.

Improved Sleep Improved Life

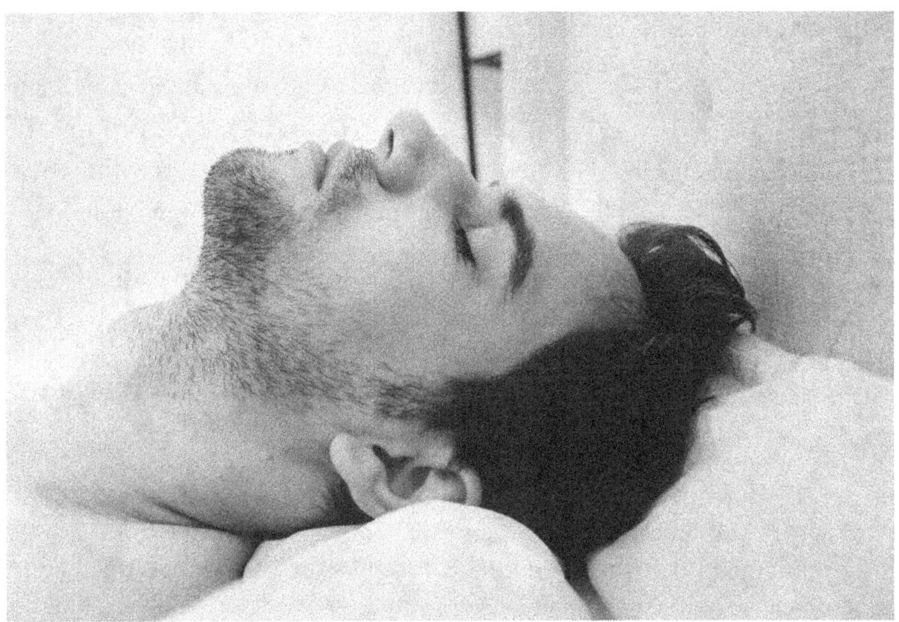

A Good Night's Sleep is an essential part of a healthy lifestyle. However, most people underrate the significance of a quality sleep. Poor quality or inadequate sleep can have a detrimental effect on your day-to-day well-being and also boosts the risk of developing health issues.

Through improved sleep, you can improve your life and overall health and wellness.

A lack of sleep can definitely ruin your next day. In due course, sleep troubles can simply wreck more than your morning mood. Various studies reveal that getting quality sleep regularly can help improve all types of health issues such as blood pressure, sugar spikes, etc.

Your improved energy is the most obvious benefit of a quality sleep that proves why sleep matters. You'll always wake up feeling refreshed after getting adequate sleep and you'll feel all set to take on the next day.

Sleep allows you to function better throughout the next day. If you get inadequate sleep, you'll find it difficult to focus or remember important things. Poor sleep eventually contributes to severe health issues such as diabetes, obesity, heart disease, high blood pressure, and cerebral disorders such as anxiety and depression.

Lack of sleep may also disrupt your hormonal balances that can lead to bad appetite control, increased fat storage, and higher stress levels. Sleep problems may also weaken your immune system that can result in frequent illnesses.

Kids also need plenty of sleep in order to perform well in studies and sports and feel their best. Lack of proper sleep will make children become more impulsive and irritable, and less attentive and sociable than their peers who get adequate sleep. This can result in lower IQ scores and bad academic performance, specifically in language skills.

Younger kids need more sleep and as they age, their sleep hours decrease. Toddlers can sleep for 10 -12 hours, school-age kids sleep for 9-10 hours, and adolescents sleep for 8-9 hours per night. To achieve these many hours of sleep, parents need to implement a regular bedtime routine at home.

Parents also can do many other things to boost their kid's energy.

They can create a relaxing sleep environment, encourage an active lifestyle, and end homework and playtime a couple of hours before sleep. Such measures can help children get their quota of quality sleep that is necessary for their overall growth and development.

3.1) How improved sleep can help improve your life?

Improved sleep can help improve your life in the following ways:

3.3.1) Sharper Brain

Sleep deprivation can affect your ability to memorize. You'll have trouble remembering things or details. Sleep plays a huge part in both memory and learning. Lack of sleep can disrupt your focus, hampering your ability to learn, and memorize new information. Sleep allows your brain to revitalize so you're ready for the next new information.

3.1.2) Healthy Heart

Your blood pressure decreases while you sleep. As a result, your heart and blood vessels get some due rest. Lack of sleep can lead to increased blood pressure that stays up for a longer period. High blood pressure may result in heart disease such as stroke.

Due to sleep deprivation, your body releases a stress hormone called cortisol that sets off your heart to pump faster. To function properly and powerfully, your heart also needs some rest. Therefore, these short-term rests while your sleep can have long-term benefits.

3.1.3) Better Mood

During sleep, your brain processes your emotions. Your mind requires some time to recognize and respond the right way. When your sleep is cut short, you tend to develop more negative emotional responses and just a few positive ones.

Chronic sleep deprivation can also increase the chance of a mood disorder. Various studies suggest that when you suffer from insomnia, your chances of developing depression are five times high. Plus, your odds of developing panic disorders and anxiety are even higher.

Good refreshing sleep helps you hit the reset button, prepares you to meet new challenges, and improves your perspective on life.

3.1.4) Athletic Accomplishment

Sleep deprivation can affect your athletic accomplishment if your sport requires rapid bursts of energy such as weightlifting or wrestling. It may also affect your performance in endurance sports such as running, biking, and swimming.

Sleep deprivation not only robs you of energy and time to repair your muscle, but it also weakens your motivation that can affect your athletic performance. You'll experience a tough physical and mental challenge that may slow your reaction times. A good quality sleep sets you up both mentally and physically for your best performance.

3.1.5) Better Immune System

A quality sleep gives your immune cells and proteins the much-needed rest to help fight off whatever germs, bacteria, and diseases come their way, such as, cold or flu. Many sleep specialists believe that good sleep can also help make medicines more effective.

To fight off diseases or illnesses, your immune system recognizes harmful viruses and bacteria in your body and obliterates them. But, sleep deprivation can severely disrupt the way your immune system functions. As a result, the immune cells may not attack the germs and bacteria in your body as swiftly as they should, and you may become ill more often.

3.1.6) Steady Blood Sugar Levels

Your blood sugar levels drop during the deep, slow-wave stage of your sleep. When you don't reach this deepest stage of sleep, you don't get that necessary break to allow a reset. Consequently, your body will have a tough time responding to your blood sugar levels. When you reach this deep sleep state, you're less likely to suffer from type 2 diabetes.

3.1.7) Weight Control

When you get sufficient sleep, you feel less hungry. But, when you are sleep-deprived, it messes with leptin and ghrelin, the two hormones in your brain, which control your appetite.

Ghrelin helps boost appetite and leptin informs your body that you're full. Sleep deprivation reduces the production of leptin in your body. When these two hormones go berserk, your resistance to the lust for unhealthy foods also goes haywire.

Lack of sleep can make you more stressed, and you'll not have the power to ward off junk food cravings. Plus, when you feel tired, you won't like getting up and moving your body. As a result, you're more likely to put on excess pounds.

To help control your weight, the time you spend at the gym and at the table goes hand-in-hand with your sleep time. Getting a full 8 hours of sleep may not directly result in weight loss, but it can surely keep your body from adding on the pounds.

We'll discuss weight control in detail, in one of my other upcoming books.

3.1.8) Increased Productivity

Postponing a good night's sleep by burning the midnight oil can have an adverse effect on your studies or work. In reality, quality sleep can help improve focus and higher cognitive function. However, one sleepless night can leave you feeling exhausted, and the chances of you committing mistakes are high that even caffeine won't be able to fix.

Speaking of caffeine, the more exhausted you feel, the more you'll crave for that cup of coffee or tea in the afternoon. And although that caffeine intake may fix your afternoon crash trouble, the additional caffeine late in the d a y   c o u l d   p r o v e counterproductive, resulting in another sleepless night.

3.1.9) Sleep Deprivation Could Be Dangerous

A study conducted by the **AAA Foundation for Traffic Safety**[20] found that instead of getting a full 8 hours of sleep, if you sleep for 6 to 7 hours, you're twice as likely to get in a road accident. If you sleep less than 5 hours, your chances of a road accident increase fourfold. The reason behind this is your response time slows way down when your brain doesn't get full rest. So, getting a full 8 hours of sleep is really necessary.

3.1.10) Increased Workout Performance

An **NCBI study**[21] was conducted on some basketball players to research the effects of sleep deprivation. The study found that the performance of the players diminished when they didn't sleep well. It clearly shows that sleep affects all kinds of sports or workout performance. Sleep recovery helps with muscle revival, reaction time, and hand-eye coordination. Sleep deprivation can have an adverse impact on your strength and power.

The bottom line: Improved sleep can improve your life because sleep is necessary. Various scientific studies reveal that those who don't get proper sleep tend to eat more, gain weight, have a higher BMI, and have higher chances to get Type 2 diabetes.

Steady sleep of 7 to 8 hours every night is a must for all adults for daytime functioning. It means being able to focus on your task, being attentive for the day, and not being tired and moody during the day.

Therefore, you should aim for getting 7 to 8 hours of sleep every night to allow your body and mind to fully reap all the benefits of sleep.

Practice In The Day To Allow An Improved Night

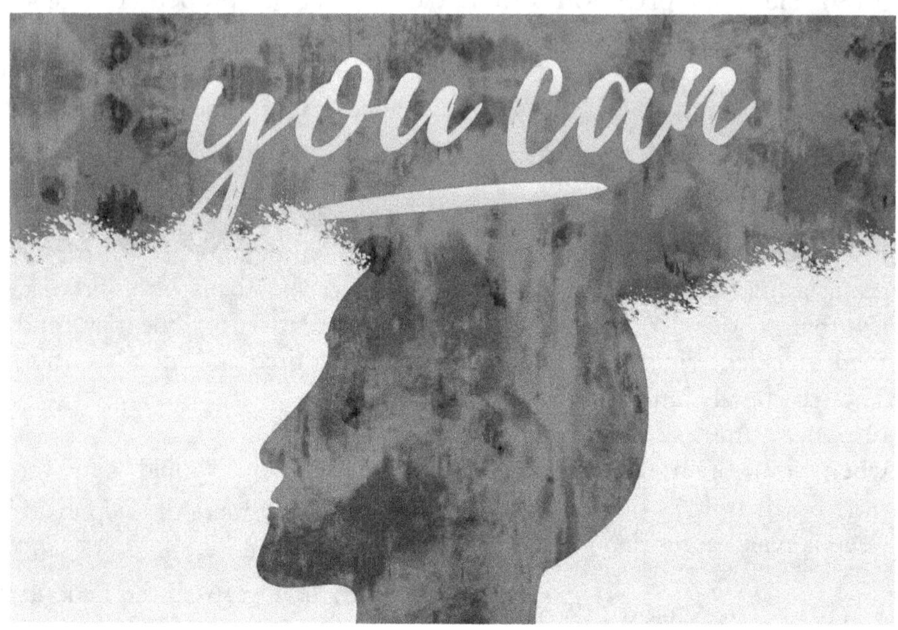

One of the best ways to train your mind for a good night's sleep is positive self-suggestion or auto-suggestion. During the daytime, start practicing auto-suggestion.

4.1) The Power of Positive Self-suggestion

Also known as auto-suggestion, this practice involves telling yourself to relax, breathe, and focus in a calm and positive manner. Using this technique, you can easily re-program your subconscious mind.

Both thought stopping and cognitive restructuring work to disrupt and change existing thought habits. On the contrary, self-suggestion techniques symbolize an effort to build new thought habits. These techniques work by way of suggestion, which means the presentation of a novel and desirable thought, image, or idea, which is repeated numerous times.

In truth, we all have used positive self-suggestion at some point in our lives. But, rather than focusing on positive things, people typically use self-suggestion to think about negative things. For example, you might say, "I am useless", "I am tired" to yourself multiple times and then wonder why you feel that way.

When you say to yourself in a doubtful, subdued voice, with a heavy, submissive feeling that "I really want to sleep well", this won't help you sleep! Always try to say positive things to yourself and feel good while doing that. Never say negative things to yourself, such as "Tomorrow will be a bad day if I don't sleep well tonight."

According to some ancient texts, your tongue possesses the power of life and death. This implies that the words you speak possess the power to either destroy or build you. So, it's better to use positive words to help create positive vibes instead of negative ones.

Where you put your focus, energy flows that way. If you say you're ugly, you'll end up being ugly. If you say you're smart and confident, your body language and appearance will exhibit it.

You can use positive self-suggestion techniques to sleep better, combat anxiety, and improve performance at work,

sport, and studies. It helps boost confidence, improve focus, feel relaxed, and remain energetic during the whole day. If these techniques are used negatively, the results can be the exact opposite.

The power of positive self-suggestion is huge. Apart from getting better sleep, you can use it for good health, career, emotional healing, deterrence, and relationships in a big way.

4.2) Self-Suggestion Techniques

Following are the top proven self-suggestion techniques:

4.2.1.) Erase negative thoughts

Start practicing positive self-talk. Whenever you find yourself doing negative self-talk, for instance, internal dialogue that conveys self-loathing, doubt, or fear, simply erase or delete those thoughts from your mind. After that, replace it with positive motivating words.

Let's say you did something wrong and you say to yourself "Why am I so stupid?" Instantly say "DELETE!" and say something motivating and positive that is apt to the situation, for example, "I've learned something important and I'm doing better and better". Don't shy away from giving yourself a direct suggestion such as "Relax", "Slow down", or "Focus".

4.2.2) Use positive affirmations

You can use positive affirmations to exploit the power of self-suggestion. Affirmations are positive and powerful sentences that you continuously repeat in your mind and heart until they're rooted in your subconscious mind, for example, "I possess the traits required to be remarkably successful."

Positive affirmations are not just some random positive statements or feel-good quotes. The word "Affirmation" stands for positive. It's a present-tense word stated in the first person. The same rules that are applicable to affirmations, you can apply them to self-suggestion techniques.

4.2.3) Use positive repetition

How many times do you say derogatory and negative things to yourself? You'll be surely surprised at the numbers. You can use positive repetition to counter this negative programming.

The self-suggestion technique involves positive repetition of a new idea, or a goal, or a purpose multiple times in a day. This technique can typically be practiced in the form of affirmations that are intended to boost self-esteem, for example, "I am a good and honest person", or team chants that are intended to boost or motivate team spirit.

However, you can repeat any positive statement as per your wish. The technique is based on learning theory. When you repeat a positive statement again and again, you condition your mind to learn that statement.

If the situation feels appropriate, you can do it out loud or you can do it silently if you need some privacy. Consider boring repetitive tasks as an opportunity to reprogram your subconscious mind with self-suggestion. Many affirmation practitioners like to practice repetitions at the bus stop, while driving, in the shower, or on a train, plane, or bus.

However, affirmation repetitions can be a tricky task. The main purpose of repeating positive affirmations is to make you believe in those affirmations. When you begin the repetition process, you actually don't believe those affirmations. Believing is a gradual process.

So, it's important that you only repeat those affirmations that you believe or you've thought about, at least at some level. You need to repeat positive truths to yourself, and avoid swallowing falsehoods.

4.2.4) Use emotions

Your self-suggestion technique ought to trigger feelings for better outcomes. It must appeal to you emotionally. The more evocative self-suggestion is to you, the more positive and effective would be the outcomes.

4.2.5) Gradual approach

Pick a quiet space to sit comfortably, for example, your home, office, or a garden. Choose an objective or purpose to focus on. Inhale long deep breaths to relax your whole body. Listen to your inner voice, and connect to the emotion that truly believes this objective or purpose. Start to imagine the accomplishment of that objective or realization of your purpose. Use all of your five senses to form a clear and detailed picture in your mind. Contemplate your objectives. Conclude with a positive affirmation about the end result of your objective or purpose.

Repeat the entire process for ten minutes, at least once a day.

4.2.6) Use Imagery

You can practice positive self-suggestion with imagery or words, or a combination of both. For example, if you are practicing weight-loss, try to put your photograph at your current weight alongside a photo of your younger (skinny) self. This can help you motivate yourself to maintain your diet and exercise regularly.

To make the imagery technique more effective, make sure to frequently look at these photos. If you simply paste them on your refrigerator or a wall, most likely you'll get accustomed to them and after a while, you won't even notice them.

Many sportspersons use imagery techniques to improve their game. For example, golfers use imagery to improve their swing. Before they actually swing their clubs, they pause to visualize themselves swinging their clubs in a perfect arc. Such imagery comprises a form of practice that helps make the real club swing more relaxed and smoother. This technique is applicable to any skill that could be improvised with practice.

You can also use imagery to help

relax and motivate yourself. When you feel relaxed, you experience good sleep.

In the next chapter, we'll discuss how to overcome blocks to a great night's sleep.

4.2.7) Use Relaxation

You can pair the relaxation technique with your self-suggestion technique to get better control of your mood states. The combination of these techniques can help create an association between specific affirmations and a serene feeling.

For instance, you can repeat words like "Relax" and "Peace" to yourself and put yourself into a relaxation state. Conversely, you can visualize a serene nature sight while relaxing.

Such images or words may not be particularly meaningful by themselves, but, in due course, with repeated pairings with the state of relaxed mind, you'll be able to set up a connection between the images, words, and emotions.

At that point, visualizing the image or repeating the words to yourself could help you enter into that relaxed state more quickly when you need to.

Overcoming Blocks To A Great Night's Sleep

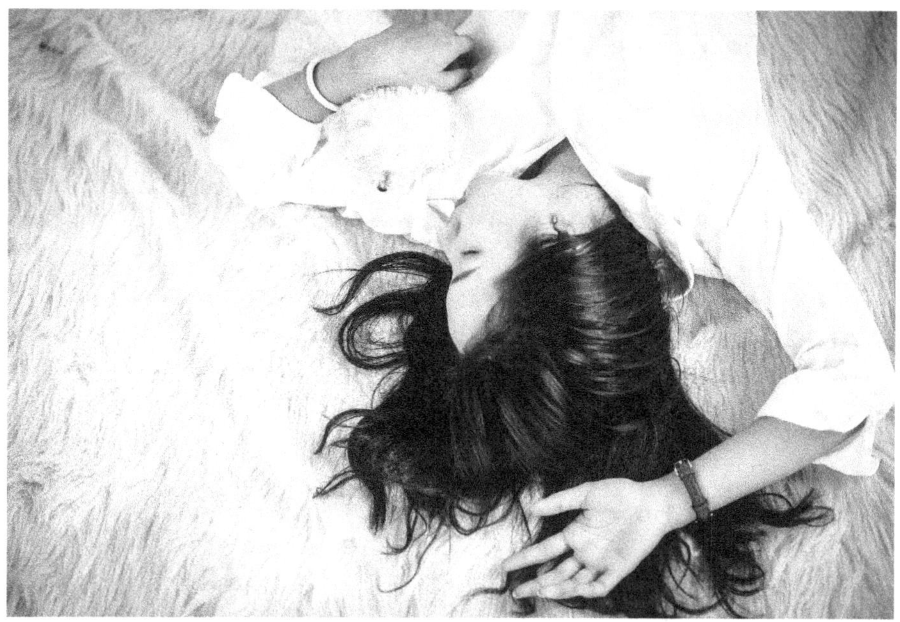

Awakeful night presents many unresolved issues. Your brain starts to buzz as soon as it's time to go to bed. You experience racing thoughts that keep gnawing at you. Such thoughts may turn into worries like not being able to properly work the next day since you slept poorly. All this can take the form of a vicious cycle.

Sleep deprivation affects your ability to sustain attention, use language, comprehend what you are reading, and recap what you are hearing. Lack of sleep can adversely affect your performance at work, your interpersonal relationships, and your mood. Therefore, getting good-quality sleep is really important.

5.1) Four pillars of quality sleep

Following are the four key factors that affect your sleep. Understanding these factors can help overcome mental blocks and heal your sleep troubles.

5.1.1) Health

Any physical health problems can disrupt your sleep. It'll be very difficult to sleep with a headache, toothache, or blocked nose. Consult your physician to treat your health problem. Avoid taking any medication without consulting your physician. If the medication isn't right for you, it can cause sleep deprivation.

Mental health issues such as depression and anxiety can also disrupt your sleep. Therapies like hypnosis and CBT can help tackle both your poor sleep and mental health issue.

5.1.2) Environment

Try to keep your bedroom distraction-free as this is the place that associates with your sleep the most. Get rid of all distractions from your bedroom. You can have your meals, play computer games, or watch TV in another room. A distraction-free bedroom is a must for a good night's sleep.

Be watchful of electronics and gadgets, such as smartphones, computers, tablets, and LED TVs. Their displays produce blue light that suppresses the production of melatonin hormone that helps in sleep. Melatonin suppression can result in sleep disruption. Stop using these electronic devices two hours before going to bed to decrease their impact on your sleep.

Some common factors that affect everyone's sleep are noise, light, and temperature. Excess noise or light can disrupt your sleep. You can use ear-plugs or eye masks if you can't control the sources of noise and light, for instance, noise from your neighbor's home or a street lamplight.

Your room temperature can also affect your sleep. Opening your window or using a thinner cover can help you sleep if the room temperature is too hot. If your room temperature gets too cold at night, you can use a thicker duvet or a heater.

5.1.3) Attitude

Lack of sleep, especially before an important day, can keep you worried. But, this worry can further disrupt your sleep.

There are many relaxation techniques that you can use to unwind yourself and relax. Also, rather than staying in bed and getting more worried, get up, and drink some water. Water will help you feel relaxed. Then, return to bed.

If your sleep troubles continue for more than a month, you could consult a professional hypnotherapist or CBT practitioner to help treat your sleep problems. Hypnosis supports a more positive attitude that can help you break the negative thoughts cycle, which causes sleep deprivation and help develop an improved sleep pattern.

Your professional Basingstoke Hypnotherapist 4 You facilitates the process and helps to produce the therapeutic change you desire.

5.1.4) Lifestyle

To improve your sleep quality, you need to maintain a healthy lifestyle and diet.

Regular workouts can help you sleep better, as well as, relieve stress and reduce anxiety. However, you need to workout at the right time. Morning workouts are considered the best. Workouts help increase the production of adrenaline in your body. If you do it just before bedtime, it'll cause sleep problems.

Consuming sleep-inducing foods such as oats, rice, and dairy products can help you sleep better. But, foods and drinks that contain high sugar or caffeine levels can cause sleepless nights. To sleep better, you need to avoid caffeinated drinks like tea, coffee, and sugary foods like chocolate late in the day.

Alcohol often messes up your sleep quality, though sometimes it can help induce sleep by making you feel tired. As the alcohol effects subside, you'll more likely wake up during the night, frequently go to the toilet, or if you feel dehydrated, you'll wake up to drink water multiple times.

5.2) Sleep disorder therapy vs. medication

Sleep deprivation causes mental and physical health problems that can tempt you to opt for a sleeping pill. However, sleep medication won't address the underlying symptoms or heal your sleep problem. On the contrary, it can worsen your sleep trouble in due course.

Therapy can prove to be more effective than medication for many sleep-related issues such as insomnia since therapy is not associated with any long-term health concerns or unpleasant side effects.

This doesn't mean that sleep medications aren't required at all. These are most effective when used in moderation for short-term situations to avoid tolerance and dependence. These short-term situations include recovering from a medical procedure or traveling across different time zones.

If prescription medication is required for your sleep disorder, medical experts would always suggest a drug regimen in combination with therapy and lifestyle changes.

We have already discussed in Chapter 2 how therapies like Hypnosis and CBT (Cognitive-behavioral therapy) can help improve your night's sleep. These therapies can help change your behavior before going to bed and change your thinking patterns that give you sleepless nights.

Therapy also focuses on altering lifestyle habits and improving relaxation skills that affect your sleeping behavior. Sleep problems typically happen due to emotional health issues, for example, stress, anxiety, and depression. Sleep problems may even trigger these emotional health issues.

Therapy can effectively treat the underlying problem instead of just the symptoms, and help you develop healthy sleeping habits for life. Therapy can help calm your mind, improve your daytime habits, transform your outlook, and prepare you for a good night's sleep.

5.3) Sleep Disorder

It's a medical condition that often affects your ability to get adequate quality sleep that leaves you feeling sleepy or worn out throughout the next day. Following is the list some common sleep disorders:

- Sleep apnea
- Insomnia
- RLS (restless legs syndrome)
- Narcolepsy
- Circadian rhythm sleep disorders (due to jet lag or shift work)

5.4) How CBT (cognitive behavioral therapy) treats sleep disorders?

CBT is the most popular therapy to treat sleep disorders. This therapy can be conducted individually, in a group, or even online. CBT could be customized to your specific problems since the symptoms and causes of sleep disorders vary significantly.

For instance, CBT for insomnia is a special kind of therapy to treat people who are not able to get the quality of sleep they require to wake up feeling refreshed.

The duration of the therapy

depends on your sleep disorder type and its severity. CBT is pretty short-term, although is rarely an easy or instant cure. For instance, many CBT programs for insomnia have shown noteworthy improvement in sleep habits in just 5 to 8 weeks sessions.

CBT tackles negative behavior and thought patterns, which contribute to sleep disorders such as insomnia. CBT involves the following components:

- **Cognitive therapy:** It helps you to identify and alter negative thoughts and beliefs that give you sleepless nights.
- **Behavioral therapy:** It helps you recognize behaviors that contribute to your sleep troubles and switch them with good sleep habits.

5.4.1) Cognitive therapy

Cognitive therapy comprises thought challenging (or cognitive restructuring) in which you confront the negative thoughts that give you sleepless nights, and switch them with more realistic, positive thoughts. By changing your thinking patterns, you can change the way you feel and eventually change your sleeping habits.

However, switching negative thoughts with more realistic, positive thoughts is easier said than done, since negative thoughts are also a part of your lifelong thinking pattern. You need constant practice to break this negative thinking pattern. So, practice the techniques that you learned in the therapy sessions whenever you get the chance at home or in the office.

5.4.2) Behavioral Therapy

Besides changing your thinking patterns, CBT also helps change your habits and behaviors that give you sleepless nights. Based on your specific needs and symptoms, your therapist may use some of the following methods:

- **Hypnosis:** During hypnosis, when you reach the deep relaxation state, your hypnotherapist uses different healing techniques to alter your negative thought patterns and perverse habits, and encourage relaxing sleep.
- **SRT (Sleep restriction therapy):** This therapy lessens your wakeful time on the bed by getting rid of naps and forcing you to stay awake past your usual bedtime. This sleep deprivation technique can be really effective for insomnia. It makes you more worn out the next night and creates a stronger bond between your sleep and

your bed, which is better than just lying awake on the bed.

- **SCT (Stimulus control therapy):** This therapy helps recognize and alter sleep habits that frequently disrupt your good night's sleep. It trains you to use your bedroom just for sex and sleep, instead of watching TV, playing computer games, or working. It also helps maintain steady sleep-wake times every day, including weekends.
- **Improve your sleep hygiene and sleep environment:** Your therapist may suggest using earplugs, eye-masks, or blocking out any noise to make your sleep environment cool, quiet, dark, and comfortable. To improve your sleep hygiene, you need to improve your daytime habits, for example, regular workouts, avoiding caffeine and nicotine late in the day, and unwinding before going to sleep.
- **Paradoxical intention:** This technique involves staying passively awake. The feeling of not being able to sleep creates anxiety in your mind that keeps you awake. So, you make no effort to sleep and you don't worry about this. It could, paradoxically, help you wind down and ultimately fall asleep.
- **Relaxation training:** Several relaxation techniques like breathing exercises, progressive muscle relaxation, and mindfulness meditation, can help relax your mind, relieve stress and anxiety, and prepare you for a good night's sleep.

Keep in mind that therapy for sleep disorders is a lengthy and gradual process. Developing good sleep habits takes time and commitment. You need to see it through if you wish to reap the benefits.

You can make positive lifestyle choices to support your therapy. It'll immensely improve your ability to sleep. Be physically active throughout the day. Workout regularly since it can help reduce stress and anxiety. A calm mind helps you sleep better. But, avoid doing workouts just before bedtime.

Avoid caffeine and nicotine at least 8 hours before sleep. Sugary foods should be avoided too since these are stimulants. Avoid alcohol since it interferes with your sleep cycle and can worsen your sleep disorder symptoms.

Tools For Successful Sleep

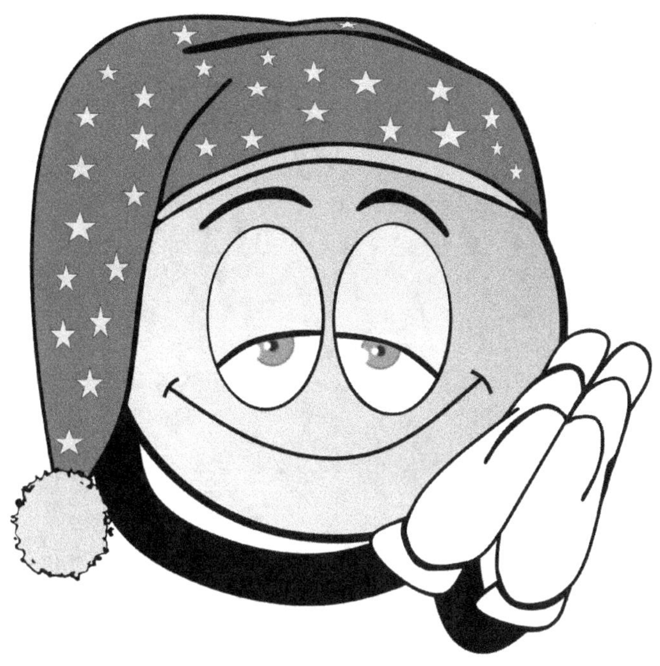

Sleep problems can really mess up your life, and it can be intricate to recognize the underlying issues and set things right.

Most probably your sleep troubles didn't develop overnight. So, give yourself the time you require to improve your sleep. Take your time to discover what works for you since different methods work for different individuals.

Non-clinical sleep disorders typically transpire due to worry and anxiety and are frequently more imagined than real. So, a good night's sleep just needs a way of stopping these worries that are hampering your sleep.

6.1) Top tools for a good night's sleep

Following are some of the top proven ways to break your old sleep habits and develop new ones:

- **Positive self-suggestion:** We've already discussed in Chapter 4 the benefits of practicing self-suggestion. This practice involves telling yourself to relax, breathe, and focus in a calm and positive manner. Using this technique, you can easily re-program your subconscious mind. When you say to yourself in a doubtful, subdued voice, with a heavy, submissive feeling that "I really want to sleep well", this won't help you sleep! Always try to say positive things to yourself and feel good while doing that. Never say negative things to yourself, such as "Tomorrow will be a bad day if I don't sleep well tonight."

- **Narrate yourself good stories:** If you tell horror stories to kids at bedtime, don't expect them to sleep well! Likewise, constantly thinking about probable future disasters and unpleasant past memories, surely can give you sleepless nights. Instead, narrate yourself good stories and the kind of dreams you'd love to experience again and again, in exquisitely fine detail, no matter whether these are true or not!

- **Speak to yourself nicely:** Pay attention to your inner voice. If the thoughts in your head have an anxious, rapid tone, this is not at all good! You need to tone it down and speak to yourself in a calm, deep, nice, comforting, and hassle-free voice, maybe with a deep "Aaaaahhh..." or an odd yawn as you unwind yourself in the bed. You'll attain immediate and convincing outcomes.

- **Progressive Relaxation Technique:** This method involves lying comfortably, focusing on your feet, and visualizing a warm, relaxed, soft, and light sensation all the way up to your ankles. Allow this feeling to spread to your knees, stomach, thighs, chest, all the way up to your head until your whole body feels good. This method allows experimenting with different waves of lightness, feelings, envisioned colors and sounds, pleasant tingling, etc.

- **Look for your best 'go-to-sleep' practice:** Ask a friend or a practitioner to help you describe how you sometimes fall asleep with ease. They can ask you questions like, "What's the last thing in your mind before you drift off to sleep? When do you know you're going to sleep quickly and easily"? Next, run this process deliberately.

- **Grant yourself some credence:** Think about your least favorite task before going to sleep, for example, cleaning the floors and sink, checking your company's balance sheet, etc. If you experience sleepless nights or you wake up in the middle of the night and find it difficult to sleep again, just get up and do that least favorite task even if it's 4.00 am. I guarantee, the next time you wake up during your sleep, you'll make a different decision.

- **Discard the 'rubbish' in your head before sleep:** Keep a pen and pad within reach near your bed. If you have loads of anxious thoughts in your mind such as "what if…" and "yes but…," just note down each worry as it crops up in your head. Then, write an action next to it that you'll take to solve that concern the next day. This will help you sleep with a calm and clear mind.

- **Relax to sleep peacefully:** As you get into bed, calm down and quietly tuck yourself in. Tell yourself "All is well", just like you would assure and comfort a child. You'll sleep safely and peacefully.

- **Program your subconscious mind:** Visualize wholeheartedly and positively, without any negative thoughts, just how well you'll feel after having your first good night's sleep. You'll feel brilliant! Then, visualize how good you'll feel after a full week of quality sleep. Then, a whole month and so on. The day will come when your sleep troubles will turn into a vague memory.

- **Develop a steady sleep pattern:** Some people have a bad habit of going to bed at different times at night. These uneven sleeping patterns could disrupt your sleep by interrupting your circadian rhythm (sleep/wake cycle). Your circadian rhythm determines whether or not your body is ready for sleep. It's heavily regulated by a biological clock that induces sleep or wakefulness by releasing hormones. Developing a steady sleep pattern can help your body clock properly anticipate when to induce sleep.

- **Avoid daytime napping:** Daytime napping can also affect your circadian rhythm. An **NCBI study**[21] revealed that students, who napped in the daytime for more than 2 hours and at least 3 times per week, experienced sleep troubles. It is tempting to take a daytime nap after a bad night's sleep. But, this can adversely affect your natural sleep cycle, so try to avoid this.

- **Avoid cell phones at bedtime:** A **study**[23] conducted on students revealed that those with sleep troubles suffered from addictive texting behavior due to excessive cell phone usage. So, avoid using cell phones at bedtime or else you'll be susceptible to sleep problems.

- **Aromatherapy:** Aromatherapy is known to stimulate relaxation and sleep. Many people use lavender oil at bedtime to get a quality sleep. A study conducted on some young adults revealed that lavender oil had a positive effect on sleep quality. The study further found that the participants felt more energetic after waking up.

- **Find the right sleep position:** The right sleep position is important for a quality slumber since it can make a huge difference in the onset of sleep. Frequent change of sleep positions can disrupt your sleep. Sleeping on your sides is considered the best sleep position if you want to experience a good night's sleep.

- **Breathing exercises:** Practicing deep breathing exercises or specific breathing patterns can help you de-stress and ward-off anxious thoughts. Using this powerful tool, you can experience a good night's sleep. One of the most popular breathing techniques is the 4-7-8 method. It involves inhaling for 4 seconds, holding it for 7 seconds, and exhaling slowly for 8 seconds. This deep, rhythmic breathing exercise can relax your mind and promote deep slumber.

- **Steer clear of e-books at bedtime:** E-books have backlit screens that make them ideal for reading in a dark room especially at bedtime. But, this could adversely affect your sleep. In a **study**[24], young adults were given an e-book or a printed book to read at bedtime. The study revealed that when the participants used the e-book, it took them longer to fall asleep. Also, they were less alert in the mornings and more alert in the evenings compared to the participants who read the printed book. These outcomes suggest that e-books can have an adverse effect on the reader's sleep.

- **Counting numbers:** Slow countdown from 100 is an old technique of inducing sleep. This technique can distract you from anxious thoughts, which eventually will induce sleep. Another factor is boredom. This method can bore you to sleep.

- **Music therapy:** Many people relax and unwind their minds by

- listening to soothing music at bedtime. Your response to music depends on your personal preference. On the contrary, music could be stimulating also and may induce anxiety and wakefulness. So, this therapy may not work for all individuals.

- **JDI (Just Do it!):** Each of the above-mentioned technique is an effective tool for a good night's sleep. These will work successfully only when you actually practice them on a regular basis. It's the DOING that works. You need to overcome the tendency of undermining things or doing things half-heartedly. A lot of anxious individuals try things once, and once they find that these work, they undermine them so that these could possibly not be helpful. Make your mind up to JDI! (JUST DO IT!)

Link and password to your hypnotic audios https://www.basingstokehypnotherapy4you.com/book-purchase-audios

Your password is bettersleep2021

Sleep deprivation can make you prone to anger and frustration. You'll also feel exhausted, confused, and a tad more emotional. This heightened emotional sensitivity can adversely affect your self-confidence since it's hard to stay positive or brave when you feel so low about yourself.

7.1) How you can feel good whenever you want

I'll share with you a very simple technique that can make you feel good whenever you want.

Close your eyes and think of those moments when you experienced pleasure, and try to gain access to that memory. Become aware of what you see, what you feel, what you hear, and what you smell and taste.

Transport all your senses into that memory to really experience the pleasure, and ramp up the feeling. Boost it further by visualizing your pleasure as a color and adding more delightful colors to your enjoyment. Spin it one way, then the other way.

Enjoy yourself making it grow. Spin it faster and faster. Confer it a sound, a taste, and even a smell making it yours, make personal.

As you go through your pleasure, touch your index finger and thumb of your left hand. This will function as an anchor. Then, release the touch right before your pleasure reaches climax.

After that, think of something else, for instance, what you had for breakfast. In NLP (Neuro-Linguistic Programming) terms it's called breaking state.

Repeat the process. Then, contemplate what you had for lunch.

Repeat the process ten times, and enjoy this easy process.

Finally, touch your index finger and thumb of your left hand to test the anchor. You'll experience the pleasure again. If you want to feel even better, start the whole process from the beginning.

This easy technique has the power to enable you to feel good whenever you want. Here's the recap:

- Choose the pleasure. Visualize (see, hear, and feel) it. Gain access to that experience.
- Touch your index finger and thumb right before your feeling reaches its peak.
- Test the anchor.
- Repeat the process if you didn't feel a strong experience.

The repetition of the process will only make the experience better and it becomes easier over time.

Have faith, enjoy the process, and you can feel good whenever you want!

7.2) How sleep boosts self-belief and vice versa?

Winners of life weren't born with exceptional confidence. They constantly flexed their confidence muscles and made it a habit.

Winners of life know that without the daily dose of confidence it'll be really difficult to get very far.

Fortunately, there are some methods that you can use to give yourself a self-belief espresso shot the moment you wake up in the morning:

7.2.1) Get rid of all your ANTs

Scientists found that ANTs (automatic negative thoughts) can be very harmful to your brain and your self-confidence. Negative thoughts can crop up in anyone's mind but the worst thing you can do is let these thoughts rattle around in your mind. This can adversely affect your sleep and spoil your next day.

Just take a few minutes in the morning to contemplate these thoughts. Once you realize that most of these negative thoughts are totally irrelevant, you'll be surprised at how fast these vanish.

7.2.2) Do positive pep-talk

After getting rid of all your ANTs, the next step is to do a self-pep talk. Stanford studies suggest that well-timed affirmations may help improve health, relationships, and education with benefits that could persist for months or even years. Attend to those great traits you possess and root for yourself. Be your biggest supporter, throughout your day speak to yourself as already a person who is relaxed and calm in all situations. Say to yourself with feeling and conviction. "I leave the concerns of the day at my bedroom door, safely boxed away; I always enjoy deep and restful sleep". When you feel good about yourself, you'll sleep better, which means your day gets better. Be your own best friend, you do deserve it.

7.2.3) Learn something new while commuting

One of the best ways to boost self-belief is to learn new skills outside your work. Studies found that learning skills such as a foreign language increase your mental satisfaction. This will boost your self-confidence and won't let any negative thoughts enter your mind. As a result, you'll experience a good night's sleep and wake up feeling refreshed. So, rather than catching Pokemon or scrolling through Instagram on the subway, try listening to a podcast on computer programming or a language guide to help boost your confidence. Better still make your own positive affirmation audio, using the tips previously mentioned. Give value to the time you have, it's in the moments positive change happens.

7.2.4) Wake up refreshed

Studies done by the **US National Institute of Health**[25] revealed that there is a correlation between sleep and your optimism and self-esteem. According to the studies, less than 6 hours of sleep can lead to lowered self-esteem and 7-8 hours of sleep can help boost your confidence.

7.2.5) Delete others from your mind

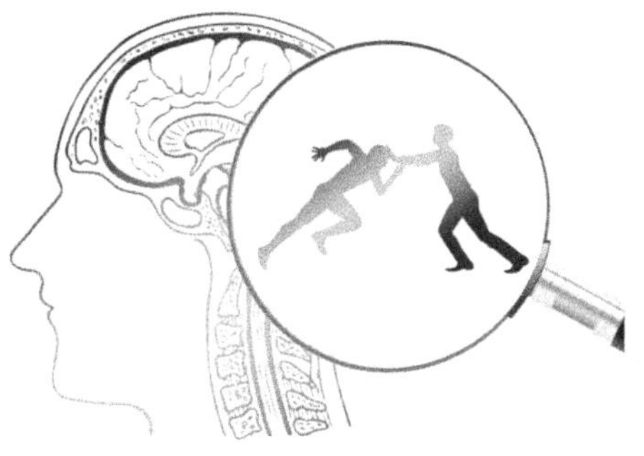

It's futile to worry about what others think of you. In truth, they seldom think of you! You're hardly a blip on their radars. Once you start to realize it, you'll stop worrying about what others think of you, and it will make you remarkably confident. You are the expert on you, no one knows you like you. No one has had exactly the experiences you have had. You are captain of your thoughts, beliefs and actions. Be your own coach.

Any lack of self-belief mainly comes from how you think others perceive you. So, begin your day by not worrying about others, even if you can't ignore your boss's opinions. You'll be surprised by the surge in your confidence. What other people think about you is none of your business.

When you incorporate these rituals, you'll be free of tensions and worries. As a result, you'll experience a good night's sleep. You'll wake up refreshed and your entire day will eventually snowball into long-lasting confidence.

Conclusion

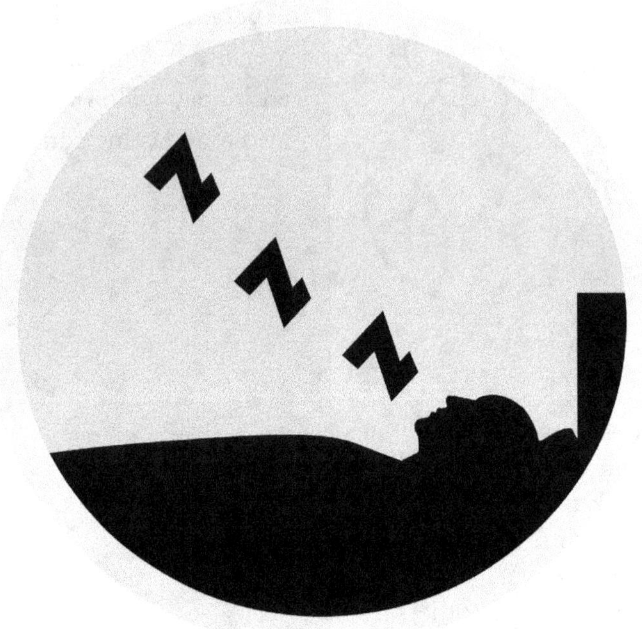

If you've reached this far, I consider this book to be worth your precious time.

It's important to eliminate stress and anxiety from your life. If the stress related to your family, school, or work gives you sleepless nights, you may have to go for stress management. To sleep better at night, you need to handle stress in a productive manner by maintaining a calm and optimistic outlook.

As a professional hypnotherapist and mind coach, I often get hundreds of queries each month from people with sleep troubles. Most of them have no idea about the root cause of their sleep problems. They often consider medication or pills as a remedy for this problem.

That's why I created this book to teach those with sleep troubles the fundamental concept and importance of sleep. This book has genuinely touched as well as explained vital topics related to sleep and sleep troubles such as the importance of sleep for your physical, mental, and spiritual well-being.

We discussed multiple techniques to train your mind to sleep faster, better and deeper including hypnosis and CBT. We covered various important topics like fundamentals of the brain, hypnosis and brain activity, the role of HPA axis in hypnosis, RAS, conscious and subconscious mind, critical faculty, and the reality of willpower.

We even discussed how improved sleep can improve your life. We also covered topics such as the power of positive self-suggestion and self-suggestion techniques.

We even discussed the benefits of hypnosis and how the hypnotic audios you NOW have access too, will really improve your sleep pattern. As you listen to them daily, the changes WILL take please. Because what you think about is what you become.

We also discussed how to overcome blocks to a great night's sleep. We talked about the four pillars of quality sleep, sleep disorder therapy vs. medication, and how CBT treats sleep disorders.

We then discussed the top tools for a good night's sleep. We also covered topics such as how you can feel good whenever you want and how sleep boosts self-belief and vice versa.

And this brings our book to an end! I sincerely believe that this book will immensely assist you in understanding sleep troubles, their root cause, and how therapies like hypnosis and CBT can help you achieve a good night's sleep with GREAT SUCCESS!

Thanks again for going through this Book and I genuinely wish you a happy and most prosperous life!

Thank You and Good Luck!

Link and password to your hypnotic audios https://
www.basingstokehypnotherapy4you.com/book-purchase-audios
Your password is bettersleep2021

[1] https://www.cdc.gov/media/releases/2016/p0215-enough-sleep.html
[2] https://www.cdc.gov/healthyschools/features/students-sleep.htm?
CDC_AA_refVal=https%3A%2F%2Fwww.cdc.gov%2Ffeatures%2Fstudents
-sleep%2Findex.html
[3] https://pubmed.ncbi.nlm.nih.gov/21172606/
[4] https://pubmed.ncbi.nlm.nih.gov/21059762/
[5] http://healthysleep.med.harvard.edu/healthy/matters/benefits-of-sleep/
learning-memory
[6] https://pubmed.ncbi.nlm.nih.gov/25861266/
[7] https://pubmed.ncbi.nlm.nih.gov/10779247/
[8] https://pubmed.ncbi.nlm.nih.gov/15576884/
[9] https://www.ncbi.nlm.nih.gov/books/NBK560713/
[10] https://pubmed.ncbi.nlm.nih.gov/29680423/
[11] https://www.health.harvard.edu/blog/mindfulness-meditation-helps-fight-
insomnia-improves-sleep-201502187726
[12] https://jamanetwork.com/journals/jama/fullarticle/189099
[13] https://www.ncbi.nlm.nih.gov/pmc/articles/PMC3630961/
[14] https://pubmed.ncbi.nlm.nih.gov/24744759/
[15] https://pubmed.ncbi.nlm.nih.gov/19488073/
[16] https://pubmed.ncbi.nlm.nih.gov/10359467/
[17] https://pubmed.ncbi.nlm.nih.gov/22525486/
[18] https://pubmed.ncbi.nlm.nih.gov/10692138/
[19] https://pubmed.ncbi.nlm.nih.gov/24860550/
[20] http://publicaffairsresources.aaa.biz/wp-content/uploads/2016/11/Acute-
Sleep-Deprivation-and-Risk-of-Motor-Vehicle-Crash-Involvement.pdf
[21] https://pubmed.ncbi.nlm.nih.gov/21731144/
[22] https://pubmed.ncbi.nlm.nih.gov/25397662/
[23] https://www.semanticscholar.org/paper/Mobile-Phone-Use-and-Sleep-
Quality-and-Length-in-Igou-White/
f742a220109064ae379a73f6c299ed1b2ca76609?p2df
[24] https://www.pnas.org/content/pnas/112/4/1232.full.pdf?
__hstc=93655746.972fdd7a7debc8575bac5a80cf7e1683.1477353600071.14773
53600072.1477353600073.1&__hssc=93655746.1.1477353600074&__hsfp=1
773666937
[25] https://pubmed.ncbi.nlm.nih.gov/23055029/